"I thought my Panic Attacks would never end, but they did!"

Contents

How to Stop Anxiety &

Panic Attacks

This book contains general reference information and is not intended as a substitute for consulting with your physician. Neither the publisher nor the author assumes any responsibility for any adverse effects that may result from your use of this book. I am not a doctor, and I do not give any medical advice in this book. If you suspect you have a medical problem, we urge you to seek medical attention from a competent health care provider.

Before We Start

Thank you for starting this special journey. While it may be difficult to imagine right now, this book will be the first domino that will start the change you've been seeking.

That's quite a statement, I know. But it's true. In this book I will show you how to stop panic attacks. It will be an amazing journey, and I hope you are excited. As I'm writing this book for you in my house in Brussels, I am very excited about the change it can initiate in your life. I've helped thousands of people overcome their panic attacks through a CD course I sell on my Web sites. One day a client sent me an e-mail stating, "Geert, you should write a book about this, too. I'm sure you'll help a lot of people with it." So that's what I did.

You'll hear stories about my clients that have already stopped their anxieties, and you may recognize yourself in some of them. Those will be the key moments in which change will happen. Realizing that you are not alone is one thing that will help, and knowing exactly what to do to get out of this situation the second secret to success.

You can only get over your panic attacks once, and the kick of being able to do the things that previously scared you will be huge. I still remember the day I realized that I hadn't had a panic attack in a couple of months—that moment was amazing. Enjoy that kick when it comes. You deserve it.

The method I'm about to explain has helped thousands of people all over the world overcome their anxieties and panic attacks, even if they had already tried EVERYTHING else.

If they can do it, you can, too.

The secret to their success is simple—dedication. In my CD course I talk about some concepts that are easy to understand but hard to apply. The same is true of this book. I'm sure you've learned by now that there isn't a magic pill that will take away panic attacks. I wish there were, but it won't happen. Instead, this book will introduce you to techniques that will not only take away you anxiety, stress, and panic attacks, but will also teach you how to enjoy every second of your life. That's why we are here in my humble opinion: to enjoy life to the fullest.

I wish you the best of luck!

Geert

P.S. I won't write an entire chapter of acknowledgements because I don't think that will help you in any way. But I do want to thank all my clients that have given me permission to publish their story in this book in the hope it would help you.

Who Am I?

And Why on Earth Should You Listen to Me?

Why should you listen to me, and why will I be the one who finally helps you after all the other things you've tried? Here's the short version of my story. It will help you, so please don't skip it.

My name is Geert, and I'm from Brussels, Belgium. I have had panic attacks (severe ones), agoraphobia, fear of driving, fear of flying, social phobia, fear of getting sick, anxiety, and stress for fourteen years. These panic attacks and anxieties limited my life to such an extent that I never left my house. That was fun.

In 2004, I finally found a solution for my problem. At first I thought I had just gotten lucky, but I still decided to try to help other people with the same problem. So I recorded everything I knew about panic attacks and anxiety on CDs and started to sell them on my Belgian Web site. The results were amazing! Within no time thousands of people had bought my CD course, and the testimonials started to come in.

That's when I expanded to other countries and languages, including English. It's not my native language, and I've actually written this book without a co-author, so don't expect any fancy words. I've refused to have this book written by a ghostwriter because I want you to get this information firsthand, which makes the information that much more powerful. What you can expect are specific techniques designed to help you with your panic attacks.

Now before you read any further, you should visit my Web site www.ilovepanicattacks.com/book/, where you can subscribe and get some additional videos that will help you with this book. You'll also find a video in which I explain my story in full.

Let's wrap this up. I'm not a doctor, and I don't have a degree in psychology. (I do have a master's degree in economics.) But I am an ex-panic attack sufferer who has apparently found a way to help you out of this.

Let's get started.

Avoidance

Fear of the Fear

- *Mike had his first panic attack while driving his car one day. This was weird to him since he loves cars and the freedom they afford. The next time he had to drive his car, he thought, "I hope I don't get another panic attack." He did and decided to avoid driving his car whenever possible.*

- *Brenda had a meal with her family at a restaurant when she experienced a feeling of warmth going through her body. She couldn't eat anymore and for some reason, she became really anxious. She wanted to get out but didn't want to upset the rest of her family. She asked to be excused and stayed in the restroom for more than thirty minutes. As of that moment, every time a suggestion was made about going to a restaurant or eating out, she found an excuse to avoid it.*

- *John had an important meeting on Thursday. He would have to give a little presentation about some projects to colleagues from another state that he'd never met. The night before he couldn't sleep. He kept going over his slides and was very nervous. The next day, he loaded up on some coffee to be alert and stay awake. Fifteen minutes before the meeting, he was a nervous wreck. He was tired and couldn't think clearly anymore. During the meeting, he had to continuously work to hide the strange symptoms he was feeling. The room was swirling around him, he had a racing heart, he was dizzy, and he could feel all the eyes that were focusing on him. He "survived" that meeting, but the entire experience was so shocking that he tendered his resignation soon afterward and searched for a job with fewer responsibilities and less pay.*

- Jenny had a stressful day at work. Before going home she stopped by the supermarket to shop for some groceries. As she was walking down the aisle with all the cleaning products, she noticed an odor that was particularly strong and unpleasant. She placed everything she needed in her shopping cart and was ready to check out. When she arrived at the checkout counter, she could see a long line of people waiting. Something was wrong with the register, and there was a short delay. While she was waiting in line, she noticed that she felt dizzy and had problems focusing on objects. Something was wrong. She started to manage herself, and she tried to calm herself down. A minute had passed and those strange sensations were still bothering her. She started to worry about all the other people. What if she fainted or if they noticed that something was wrong with her? Five minutes into her panic attack, Jenny decided to leave her cart in the checkout line and head for the exit. As of that moment, she only went to a supermarket with a friend or her husband and even then, she would feel very anxious. This wasn't an ideal situation.

These are stories of some of my clients; they all recovered and now live the lives they deserve. What's clear here is that they all encountered a very anxious period at some point; sometimes it was a panic attack, and sometimes was generalized anxiety. But the experience was so bad that they really wanted to avoid it in the future. That's how the fear of the fear is born. To avoid those symptoms and to avoid the fear, they start to limit their lives and start living in a comfort zone that gets smaller every day. This is because the anxiety will continue to find them and will spread like a little devious virus.

For me it started during a family dinner, and then expanded to restaurants, movie theaters, meetings, and driving my car. Eventually I wasn't even safe in my own bed—there simply was no safe place left. That's okay. I'm glad it became that bad because it gave me the motivation to say NEVER AGAIN and to I find a way out.

I don't know what led you to read this book, but believe me, the deeper you are in this mess now, the better your chances of getting out. You'll need that motivation to work on yourself and on your life. Avoiding situations, people, and experiences is not the solution. The anxiety will find you despite your best efforts. The real solution is learning how to play with the danger in such a way that the fear of the fear is taken away. When you'll arrive at that point, you will be able to do everything again, and you'll actually enjoy it. I'll show you how to get there.

What's Wrong with You?

Why Do You Have Panic Attacks?

Mary is forty-three years old, and she has two lovely children and a nice husband. The last couple of years, Mary has not been happy anymore. She's living her life, but she's not enjoying it. Whenever she's in a shopping mall, she wants to leave. Mary doesn't understand why, but she gets anxious even thinking about a space like that.

Driving the kids to school has become harder also. She tries to avoid the freeway because she can't get off when she wants to leave. Lately, traffic lights have become a problem, too. The problem is spreading. So she decided she doesn't want to drive at all anymore, since every road trip is a major risk for herself, and the people in the other cars.

Her career is suffering badly because of this. Mary had big dreams for herself, but she finds it hard to sit in meeting rooms. During meetings, she just wants out and often starts to feel dizzy, with a racing heart and some nausea on top of it. Her boss has already warned her that she needs to do something about it because this can't continue.

Every little part of Mary's life made her anxious. The minute she woke up, she was already thinking "what if...," and she dreaded the things she had to do that day. Her physician prescribed some antidepressants, but they only made her anxiety worse. She needed something else. There was something wrong with her, and it was imperative that she found out what it was.

That's the day that Mary decided it had to stop, and she would do ANYTHING to get out of it. Her kids deserved a better mom; her husband deserved a wife he could actually take out and have fun *with. Their last vacation or little trip was more than fifteen years ago.*

Mary heard about me from her counselor, so she visited www.ilovepanicattacks.com to see what I could do for her. She decided to use my help and started to work on herself. Three weeks later, I received an e-mail describing her first victory. Her professional performance had improved in such a way that her boss actually gave her a promotion. Seven weeks into the course, she e-mailed me that everything had changed; she still had work to do, but her life was not limited by anxiety anymore. She started to live by my mantra: Whatever happens — it is okay.

As I write this book, it's almost four years after I received that first e-mail, and Mary is still doing great.

Why do you have panic attacks? Do you honestly know?

There are many reasons, but it always comes down to two things:

1.   The way you see the world and the things you say to yourself (your inner voice or inner dialogue).

2.   Your body that communicates to you what it likes and doesn't like.

These are truly the only two causes. I don't know what you are afraid of, but whatever you fear (i.e., driving, dying, being amongst other people, finding no way out, or being alone), it is not the people you are with or the thing you are doing that is causing the anxiety or the panic attacks, it is you.

That's tough, I know. But the good news is that if you are causing it, YOU have the POWER to STOP IT. I will show you how.

If you've had a medical checkup and everything is okay, there truly is nothing wrong with you. (If you haven't had a recent checkup, you should.) Your body might be giving you very weird sensations that scare you even more, but that's all part of the panic attack system.

The Panic Attack System

Panic attacks are essentially a self-defense mechanism of our bodies. It is part of the fight-or-flight mechanism. If you and I were walking in the woods, and all of a sudden we noticed a real tiger in front of us. What would happen? Just imagine standing in the woods with a tiger that has giant teeth standing in front of you. Might it be possible that you would experience the following symptoms?

- anxiety
- racing heart
- face and skin become redder

- sweating
- faster breathing
- digestion stops
- feeling of warmth throughout the entire body
- some dizziness or vertigo

That is exactly what would happen, isn't it? Have you ever felt any of these symptoms before? Perhaps while having a panic attack?

In the woods, with that hungry tiger in front of us, we would get all of these symptoms to prepare our bodies for a major fight, or a very fast run away from that tiger. Our muscles would need extra oxygen, so our heart would start to pound faster. Our digestion would stop because that wouldn't really be important in escaping a tiger (this can result in nausea or other intestinal problems). We would breath faster to get more oxygen in, and we might get dizzy and get all kinds of weird sensations in our body, but we wouldn't care. We're not going to look at each other and say, "Hey, is there something wrong with me? I feel so weird!" Nope, that won't happen because there's a tiger standing in front of us, and he's thinking about the delicious meal before him.

What happens when you're driving your car, waiting in line somewhere, or simply minding your own business at a certain location and all of a sudden you feel these symptoms and sensations? If you're like the old version of me, you might think, "What's wrong here? Why am I feeling this? Not again. I really have to control this now! Where are the exits, and how can I get out of here? When and if you think this, it will be a panic attack or at least a very uncomfortable feeling. Let's quickly analyze why.

What type of phrase is *not again* or *what's wrong with me?* These are anxious phrases. When you think them, you are scaring yourself. This is in fact one example of how your inner dialogue (the things you say to yourself) can actually make you anxious and cause a panic attack.

When you see a tiger in front of you, you think, "Wow, a tiger! This is dangerous," and you push the panic button in your body. That's okay because there is a tiger. When you think, "What's wrong with me? Why am I so anxious?" you also push the panic button in your body, and it will launch the exact same system, with the same symptoms like the racing heart, sweating, vertigo, and fast breathing. So what you say to yourself when you're anxious will be really important, and we'll work on that in the next couple of chapters.

To recapitulate:

You've learned that your thoughts can cause a panic attack or an anxious feeling.

But there's more.

Sometimes you get these thoughts because your body is giving you certain symptoms. When you feel them, you might worry about them and become anxious.

I suffered a lot from this. I still remember sitting in a movie theater, and the commercials were running, but I could see the entire screen moving—not what was on the screen but the screen itself. I was dizzy and very nauseated. Then I started to sweat, and my heart started to beat very fast. It was so scary that I began looking for an exit and wondering how long I could keep sitting there without fainting or dying.

Restaurants were fun, too. Quite often, the minute I had my first bite I became nauseated, and my stomach would communicate DO NOT EAT ANYMORE. So I would then think, "If I stop now, what are people going to think? Maybe I need to go to the restroom?" Since I this often happened, I always wanted to sit in a place where I could see the exit and the restrooms, and I wanted to be sure nobody could sit or stand in my way if I had to get out.

In my car I had that dizzy feeling; an out-of-body experience in a way, and I continuously wondered when I would lose control of the car.

On top of all this, I was plagued by frequent headaches (real migraines) and the nausea was occurring everywhere and every time I went out.

I thought I was sick; I thought something was really wrong with me. At that time, I think it was 2002, I saw the doctors in the E.R. more than I saw my own parents. Every possible test was done on me. CAT scans, cameras in my stomach, blood testing—the works. My health was perfect; there was nothing to be found. It was clear to the doctors that it was all in my head. I was imagining thing That was what my friends told me, as well. I was creating these feelings and symptoms with my thoughts. If only I could use that power to move objects or "see" the lottery numbers before the draw.

Can you relate to my story? With all the experience I have now, I can tell you my friends and family were both wrong and right. I wasn't creating the symptoms with my thoughts—something else was. But I was making it worse. I'll dig deep into the causes of some of these symptoms later in the book.

When our body tries to communicate something by giving us a feeling, we need to accept that feeling. I made the mistake of starting to worry a lot about those feelings or symptoms and consider phrases like *What is wrong with me? Why am I having this? Oh my, please not now.* These phrases made me push the panic button.

So here are the two ways you can fire up a panic attack:

1.   **ANXIOUS THOUGHT** > ANXIOUS FEELING > MORE THOUGHTS > PANIC ATTACK

2.   SYMPTOM > **ANXIOUS THOUGHT** > ANXIOUS FEELING and MORE SYMPTOMS > MORE THOUGHTS > PANIC ATTACK

Here's an example:

1. What if I want to get out of here? I really can't because I'm not supposed to leave. Oh no, my heart is racing, and I'm getting black spots in front of my eyes. Am I going to faint? I should get out of here.

2. Why am I so dizzy? What if I want to get out of here because I'm dizzy? I really can't because I'm not supposed to leave.

Each and every time that something scares you, no matter what, you push the panic button.

Some phrases will push the button slightly—Oh, this is a funny symptom I'm feeling. Others will push the panic button very hard—Oh my, am I going to die?" The panic attack will be tied to the severity of the alarm level. The important issue here is that you and only you cause the panic attack, and only you will be able to stop it. That is good news in my opinion. You don't need anyone else or anything. You only need yourself and the way you talk to yourself.

Please rest assured that no matter what you are feeling, if the doctors have told you that you are in good health, you are. It's just the self-defense system of your body that needs to be tuned again. You will learn how to do that in a later chapter by reprogramming your mind. This reprogramming will be important. Do you remember the stories about avoidance? You get a panic attack somewhere, and then you start to avoid those things; you may prefer not to do them and sometimes you find excuses not to go somewhere or do something. That's also a part of the panic attack system.

If we did indeed meet a tiger in a certain forest, we would run for our lives in that forest. What are the chances that we would ever go back there again? That possibility is very small. And even if we were brave and returned, the moment we set foot in that same forest, we would start getting the symptoms of a panic attack. How is that possible? The reason is simple. Our body knows the danger there, and it will always do everything it can to keep us alive, so it is going to make us afraid. Even before meeting the tiger again, it is going to give us all the fight-or-flight symptoms, just in case.

This sounds like a great system doesn't it? In that type of forest situation, it would really help us. Unfortunately this also means that if you ever had an anxious feeling in a plane for instance, your body is going to scare you when you simply think about flying. It does this…just in case.

Your body and mind have been programmed to scare you whenever you come near the thing or place where you had a panic attack or a severe anxious feeling before. The emotions during an anxious moment are so strong that it is almost immediately engraved in our memories and self-defense system.

Reprogramming that system is a major part of the solution. It will not be easy; I have to be honest here, and I don't want to give you false hope. But it is possible, and that's what we are going to do in this book and in the extra videos you can watch on www.ilovepanicattacks.com/book/. If you haven't visited that site to watch some videos, please do. They are really important and part of this solution.

What Is NOT Causing the Panic Attacks

Over the years, a lot of my clients have told me what they thought were the causes of their panic attacks. Let me go over a couple of them, so we can wipe them off the table. Focusing on them is a waste of time.

The Past

I respect psychologists and therapists a lot. I think I was unlucky when I met mine. They all wanted to dig in my past. For hours I had to talk about my childhood, about experiences I've had, and so forth. That's great because indeed my panic attacks started in the past, and there were causes to be found in the past.

But those causes are in the past. They cannot be changed now, and they weren't what was keeping the anxiety alive these days. I don't like to dwell on the past, so it will not be a part of the solution I'm about to uncover for you.

What is true is that you had your first panic attack or anxious moment in the past, and your body and mind remember it. Every time you come into the same or a similar situation, you'll feel anxious. This is normal, and it's just your programming, your wiring.

Places and Locations

My panic attacks were specifically occurring in places where I couldn't get out, especially when there were people in that place (i.e., restaurant, meeting, highway, concert, or supermarket). So I started to avoid those locations. I thought they were the cause of my problems, and my theory was if I avoid these places, I will be fine, and the panic beast won't harm me anymore."

I was wrong.

I quickly found out that it wasn't a specific location since I started to experience panic attacks in my own house. Sometimes it was when I saw a movie where the characters were in a restaurant for instance, and other times I was simply reading a book in my own bed.

The places, locations, or people are not the cause. Your body has linked the panic attacks to those things and that's why you might feel anxious there. The more you try to avoid those locations or things, the worse it will get since you will actually tell yourself, "You're right. These places ARE dangerous."

About a month ago I saw a movie that included following a man into a meeting. During that meeting, we can hear his thoughts, and we can tell he's getting very nervous. He loosens his tie a bit and starts to sweat. "I need to get out of here," he says to himself. He asks to be excused and leaves the room. A couple of feet down the hallway he leans against a wall and starts to calm down. He was out of that meeting room, and all was fine. Isn't that a little bit strange? He's just two feet away and that place would be safer than the meeting room itself?

It isn't. What's going on here is the power of the inner dialogue. "I need to get out of here" scares him. He's telling himself that the meeting room is bad (for whatever reason: the people in it, the fact that he's not supposed to leave, etc.) and the hallway is safe. And guess what—because he told this to himself, it will be his truth. Once in the hallway, he will have escaped the danger and will be fine.

Most people with severe panic attacks prefer to stay home. That is their safe place. Every time they had a panic attack before, they told themselves, "I need to get home where I will be okay." Once home, they are better because that's what they told themselves.

This brings me to another very important fact:

Everything you say to yourself will always be the truth. Always.

And I'm not only talking about panic attacks here although that's what I'll focus on for now. Mike, the man in one of the examples who had a panic attack in his car, could have told himself "I'm not afraid of this car, and everything is fine here. I don't need to get out, whatever happens—it's all okay."

He wouldn't have had a panic attack. The truth is this is easier said than done, but I'll show you how to do it.

For now, please remember that you don't need to avoid anything. Those things are not causing the panic attacks or the anxiety. Your inner dialogue and your body are. This is good news because it means you can learn to control yourself wherever you are.

For now, whenever you are anxious, try to monitor that inner dialogue, the things you say to yourself. Simply try to notice it because the words and phrases that you are using will make you more or less anxious.

Your Parents or Family

When I first started to help people with anxiety and panic attacks, I met Michelle. She was convinced her panic attacks would stay with her forever. Her grandparents and her mother had experienced panic attacks, and now she had them. She was afraid her daughter would get them too.

Are panic attacks hereditary?

In my opinion, they are not. If you've joined the Web site (www.ilovepanicattacks.com/book/), you will soon get a video in which I tell the story of Bob the spider. I'll quickly go over this story to prove my point.

Little Mikey is crawling around in the living room. He's looking for his teddy bear but can't find it. "Maybe it's there, in that dark hole under the fireplace? It looks like a cave, and bears sleep in caves right?" Mikey might say to himself. So he crawls toward that dark hole and sticks his arm in it.

In the back he feels something furry. It's not Teddy, his teddy bear, because it's way too small. "Maybe it's another toy?" says Mikey to himself, so he pulls the furry thing out. He looks at it and sees it's alive. It has eight boney legs and a furry, round core. It's a funny little thing because it tries to run away every time he touches it.

Little Mikey continues to play with it for a couple of minutes. Then his mother enters the room.

"MIKEY!" she screams. "MIKEY get out of there!" She quickly pulls him away. "BRIAN, BRIAN, there's a spider in the living room. Please come and kill it—hurry!" she screams anxiously.

Mikey is in shock, and he doesn't know what's going on. He sees that his mother is very anxious, and he knows it has something to do with that furry little thing he was playing with. As of that moment, whenever Mikey sees a spider, he will become anxious. He doesn't know why. It just happens.

Do you think this is a credible story? Do you still remember how you played with certain insects when you were little? How you were not afraid of certain things but then became afraid of it because your parents were? As kids and even as adults, we are like sponges as we take in what's going on around us.

Michelle, the woman with anxious grandparents and an anxious mother was anxious because she inherited her mother's worldview. Her mother had inherited that worldview from her parents and so on. It's not in their genes; it's in what they've learned from each other Their worldview is shared. What that view is will be the topic of one of the following chapters because it really is that important. How you view the world can give you anxiety or take it away.

Being a Highly Sensitive Person (HSP)

I could write an entire book about this subject. I'll introduce you to Jennifer, just in case you don't know what a HSP is.

Jennifer always knew she was sensitive; she saw the world in a different way than most of her friends. For starters, she was very empathetic. She could get into people's minds, and she knew how they felt and what they were thinking (about her). When she had to let someone down by using the word no, *she felt guilty.*

When she was at a concert, all the people and all that noise…it was too much for her. Her body was sensitive as well, and whenever she drank alcohol, she would feel its effects much more quickly than the people she was with. When she had a cold or something minor, it always felt like a major disease. She was sensitive in every possible way and needed a lot of time alone to recharge her batteries.

Jennifer also suffered from stress, anxiety, and panic attacks, and she became agoraphobic because of all this. Her house, where she could stay away from a lot of stimuli, was a good place to be. Secretly, however, she wanted more from her life. When she followed my CD course, she found the life she wanted. For more information about my course, please visit ilovepanicattacks.com.

I don't have a magic ball that tells me everything, but I believe you probably recognized yourself a little bit in this story if you suffer from anxiety yourself.

I was an HSP, and I still am. This doesn't mean it causes anxieties because I've been living without them for a long time by now. HSP means that you are prone to anxiety and panic attacks. It's easy to get the attacks because every little symptom will feel like something bad; every little tiger will become a big tiger. Once you learn how to manage yourself, you'll see that HSPs have an advantage.

"Normal" people have fun, but they do not become ecstatic. Good things don't make them really happy, and bad things don't make them really sad. HSPs are different. Little things can make them extremely anxious, bad things can make them feel really bad, and sad but good things can make them enjoy life more than other people. That's the good side of the coin. The moment that an HSP learns how to control his or her emotions a little bit, amazing things will happen. I will show you how.

Chemical Imbalances in the Brain

Before I start this part, I want to remind you that I'm not a doctor. But doctors have told me in the past there were imbalances in the chemicals in my brain. That's what was causing the panic attacks, and therefore, I should take prescription medication.

Great. The only problem for me was the prescription meds actually made me a lot more anxious. In my personal, nonmedical opinion the medications merely hide the symptoms, without taking the causes away. For me, they tried to hide the original symptoms by giving me an avalanche of side effects. What a concept.

I'm sure there can be imbalances in the brain. If you lack serotonin, you will feel different for instance. But there are natural ways to change this and although I'm not a doctor, I'll point out some of these later on in the book, especially in the chapter about foods and sports.

The Friend Method

A First Method to Stop Panic Attacks, Anxiety, and Stress

In this book I will share a couple of techniques with you that are very effective against anxiety, panic attacks, and stress. Let me start with a powerful but simple one called the friend method.

Imagine your best friend coming to you with a problem. Let's say your best friend is sitting next to you in the car and says, "I feel very anxious, my heart is racing, and I feel dizzy. What's wrong with me?" You look at your friend, and you see the fear in her eyes (let's suppose it's a girl). What are you going to say? Will it be "Oh my gosh, you're right. Something really bad must be happening to you, and you can't get out of here since we're driving. With all these other cars around us, I can't just leave the highway. If I stop now, they would probably crash into us and…"

Would you say that? No, of course not because it sounds completely ridiculous. Well, why would you talk to yourself in such a way? Have you ever said things like that to yourself? Have you told yourself that things will go wrong or that you cannot get out or anticipated something bad happening with "what if?" phrases? I sure did that a lot.

And I still believe it's funny that we sometimes treat ourselves that way. Sometimes we treat our friends and family better than we treat ourselves. This will be a recurring theme throughout this book, but let me tell you something important:

You are the most important person you will ever meet.

It's true. You've been there from the first second, and you'll be there at the last second as well. You will always have yourself with you, and you can always rely on yourself.

I'm not fooling you here; I realize how weird this sounds, but the only person that will never ever betray you in any way is *you*. Try to think about this when you talk to yourself. Treat yourself better than you would treat your friends.

All right, back to your friend in the car. What would you say to her? You might say something to calm her down, to relax her, and although it won't take her anxiety away, it will not make it worse. The trick here is to keep those thoughts in mind when you talk to yourself when you feel anxious. This however is more complex than it seems. Let me elaborate a little.

Have you noticed already it is easy to comment on someone else's life? It's easy to tell someone else what to do. It just seems so clear.

Have you ever given anyone any relationship advice? If you have, it probably seemed so clear what they had to do. However, when you were in the same situation yourself, everything was probably different. You had all these feelings and emotions that made it difficult to see what to do. Might I be on to something here?

This emotional filter that makes it "different" because it is about you and not about someone else is the only hurdle you will have to take if you successfully want to use the friend method.

I'll start by explaining the method, and then we'll cover the challenges you might face with it.

The Friend Method

1. You get an anxious thought, you start to worry about something, and your experience has shown this might give you a panic attack.
2. You think, "Okay, my best friend comes to me and explains exactly what I'm feeling now. What would I say to this friend? Oh, I would say this and that and…"
3. Now say to yourself what you would tell your friend to help her calm down; avoid phrases like *oh my, what is going on*.

This method is just an appetizer. There are stronger things you can do against anxiety; nevertheless, this can be really powerful, so please write it down somewhere.

The Challenges You'll Face with this Method.

There are a couple of challenges. First, when in panic, when anxiety is already high, you might not find the time to imagine what you would say to a friend. So you need to prepare beforehand.

After you've had a panic attack, take a piece of paper and write down what you felt and what you thought during the attack. Try to do this as soon as you can after the panic attack, even if it's just scribbled on a scrap of paper. When you have more time, review what you wrote and apply the friend method to it. Take your time to imagine a friend coming to you and saying exactly what you were feeling. Then write down your reaction to that friend. Memorize that reaction, and the next time you feel anxious, use that as your inner dialogue.

Challenge number two is that your inner voice will say, "Yeah, but this situation is different." It really isn't. If it's what you would tell a friend, it should be what you tell yourself right now. This will calm you down, but you will need to practice with it.

I'll give you a more powerful method later that is for advanced users. Please take the time to experiment with this method now. It will be the necessary base for what is about to come.

The Way You See the World and Try to Control It

Why This Causes Stress and Anxiety

This is in fact one of the most important chapters of this book. It all begins here, and it all ends here.

How *do* you see the world? Let's do a little test. I'll give you some statements, and you respond with a number between one and five. One will stand for I'm totally not like that, three, I am like that sometimes, and five, that's me!

The Little but Important Quiz

1.   **I want everything to be under my control because otherwise I feel nervous or anxious.**

Score: *3*

2.   **I want to be liked by everyone.**

Score: *5*

3.   **When I do something, I need it to be perfect.**

Score: *3*

4.   **I want people to be fair to me.**

                  5

Score:

5.   **In relationships (friends, love, and family), I often get upset when the other person doesn't do what I want.**

                  3

Score:

6.   I want to be in perfect health at all times. No aches, no pains, and no special symptoms.

Score: 5

7.   When I have an upcoming event, I plan ahead and imagine what it will be like.

Score: 3

8.   I worry about losing control of myself, my thoughts, or my actions.

Score: 3

9.   I get irritated when things don't go as planned.   3

Score:

10.   When I know I cannot control something and when other people are in control, I feel anxious.   3

Score:

Global Score: 26

If your score was ten, I'm not sure why you are reading this book. My guess is that your score was actually higher. If your score was between ten and twenty-nine, you probably have mild anxiety and more than moderate amounts of stress that frequently disturb you.

If your score was above thirty and below forty, you will have anxious feelings quite often. You will have a panic attack here and there that will limit the fun you have in life.

If your score was fifty, I welcome you to the club I was the head and president of until 2004. I have since resigned, but I can tell you, club members have panic attacks, generalized anxiety disorder, social phobia, and all other possible anxiety-related problems. All of this is free; it really is a great club of which to be a member.

My guess is that if you are reading this book for yourself, you've scored above thirty-five. That's okay; it is no accident, and we will work on these things. Let's go over these items now and discuss why they can cause panic attacks, anxiety, and stress. Before I do, let's remember that:

An anxious thought, even a little one, can start the panic cycle.

Number one was I want everything under my control because otherwise I feel anxious or nervous.

It is actually impossible to have everything under your control and to be the master of everything, so unforeseen things cannot happen. A person who could do this would rule the world and probably the universe. Such a person doesn't exist. People who try to achieve the impossible can get tired, depressed, and anxious because they keep failing. The expectations here are simply way too high and can never be met; this gives that person a feeling of helplessness.

~

One of the worst feelings or emotions you can give yourself is when you realize you cannot control something that you need to and want to control.

~

One of the most calming emotions you can give yourself is realizing it is okay to let go of control, to let things flow, and just see what happens.

~

More on that later, but for now, it is important to know that a person who wants to control everything is wearing down his nervous system, making it so sensitive that every little thing becomes a stressor or an anxiety starter.

Number two was I want to be liked by everyone. This brings me to the story of Belinda.

Belinda is a forty-three-year-old woman; she has no children and has been divorced for seven years. Although Belinda is a social person, she has some problems in that area.

Let's take the little party she organized last Sunday as an example. It was her mother's birthday, and she and her sisters decided to host a little party for family and friends. Belinda wanted it to be perfect because her mother only turned sixty-five once, and it had to be an experience she would never forget.

Belinda was stressing about the details a couple of weeks before the party. It was as if she was planning the perfect wedding. A couple of days before the birthday, she was a nervous wreck. She couldn't sleep, she couldn't focus on anything, and she became really anxious. All those responsibilities were too much.

On Sunday, her mother's birthday, Belinda was really upset when the cake was delivered one hour late; she apologized to the guests and to her mother, and blamed her sisters, although she didn't say anything about it to them. That night, she was completely depleted and felt depressed.

Can you feel that Belinda wanted to be liked by everyone? I admit that it isn't very clear in this story of my client, and that's why it is important.

Belinda wanted to be liked by her mother. She had always been looking for her approval and fighting with her sisters for her mother's attention. During the party, she subconsciously wanted every guest to compliment her, and she wanted to make sure that everyone enjoyed the best party ever. She wanted her mother to come to her and thank her for the best day ever. This is another example of trying to control the uncontrollable.

One of the more obvious examples is the story of Frank.

When I met Frank, he was in serious trouble. At least, that's what he thought. His wife was about to leave him, and none of his friends really liked him. This was a big issue because all Frank ever wanted was to be liked.

Let's take a look at the relationship he had with his wife. She was a dominant person, and Frank was looking for her approval by doing things for her. The word no was not in his vocabulary, and his wife could literally walk over him, as could his kids. Since he decided he wanted to be a perfect father, he made sure they could never dislike him because he denied them something or punished them when they were bad.

It was the same story with his friends. He was always there for them, answering the call to help whenever help was needed. And when Frank needed help, and they declined, he kindly understood. They were busy people.

Frank is a so-called "nice guy" who tries to please everyone and keep everyone as a friend. Everyone loves Frank, but nobody respects Frank and nobody is IN LOVE with Frank. This was tough for him to hear when I first explained it to him, but it was the first step out of this situation.

When I met Frank, his wife was about to divorce him since she couldn't love a man who was such a pushover. Frank has now regained his confidence. He also added the word no to his vocabulary and has new friends that respect him.

Can you feel what's going on here?

Many people want to be liked because it's in our nature. But too much of this can turn against you and start to harm you and your relationships. When you meet people, you can *never* control what they think of you. Some people will be inclined to dislike you, others will have a neutral feeling, and others will like you. When you look at a famous person like a president, you will always see these three groups of people — the lovers, the haters, and the disinterested. This is beyond your control. There are techniques to *win friends and influence people* (see the book written by Dale Carnegie), but that falls outside of the scope of this book.

Frank and others try to win friends by pleasing them, by always being there for them, and by never ever using the word *no*. Sure, people will stick around, as long as they can use Frank. The minute he says no or the minute he's of no use, he gets dropped. You might have seen people do this to you before. I know I have. That's why they say you quickly find out who your real friends are when you are the one who needs help.

Don't waste your time on wanting to be liked. Go with the flow, be yourself, and see who sticks around. Those are the people who really love and respect you. Those are the people you should invest your time in since they are really worth it. You'll get a great return on investment there.

On a side note, when your panic attacks and anxiety are gone, you will be a new and improved version of you. The not-so-real friends will then show their true colors when they see that you don't need them anymore since you depend on yourself and not them. Don't be alarmed when this happens.

Even family members might respond in a special way when the new you doesn't "need" them anymore. Those who really love you will quickly turn around, so please don't worry about this if it should happen.

Number three was when I do something, I need it to be perfect. This is all about expectations and goals. "What if I won't make it?" is an anxious thought and is enough to give you an anxious feeling in the stomach.

Other people need everything to be perfect. Examples are:

- A clean house at all times.
- Kids raised by perfect parents.
- Be a person with no flaws.
- When they finish a project, it needs to be done as if superman himself did it.
- When going on vacation, the weather needs to be perfect.
- They want to be liked by everyone and want to be the perfect friend, significant other, parent, employer, or employee.

Feeling like a failure when they cannot reach these goals can obviously induce depression. How high do you raise the bar for yourself, and what is your reaction when you don't make it?

Anthony Robbins (a motivational speaker who coached people like Bill Clinton) taught me a valuable lesson about ten years ago. **"As long as you try, you cannot fail,"** he said. It's the minute that you stop trying that you can fail. Please notice that nothing was said about the result. It is far less important.

The people who make it in life are quite often people who set goals and try to reach them but accept when this cannot be done. They just dust themselves off and try again and again and again.

I don't know you personally, but my guess is although your expectations might be too high, you still are someone who keeps trying. I'm sure, for instance, that this book isn't the first thing you've tried for your anxious feelings. Anthony Robbins helped me out a lot specifically with this part; don't underestimate these high expectations because they can cause panic attacks and anxiety. The whatever happens—it is okay technique I'll talk about later will work great in this area.

As a little exercise I invite you to take a piece of paper and write down the expectations in your life. I mean both what you expect of yourself and what others expect of you.

This second point, mixed with a desire to please other people, can obviously be very dangerous. The mere fact that you identify these things with this exercise is the first step out of this stress and anxiety. Remember, YOU are the most important person you will ever meet. No matter what anyone else wants from you, you should always decide if it is what you want or not.

On a side note, I want to emphasize that happy people who make it in life do set goals, and they try to reach them. The big difference is they don't get upset when they don't achieve them; they just try again. Think of people like Donald Trump who have rebounded from bankruptcy or movie stars who don't always get a call back after an audition. For every role we see them play, they've gotten turned down hundreds of times before.

Someone once said It's better to aim for the stars and miss than to aim for the mud and make it. It's what you do when you miss the stars that defines you. Take it with an attitude of okay. Lesson learned. I'll try a new way to reach this, and your stress level will go down so much that it will actually become easier to reach your goals.

Life will not always be perfect; we all have rainy days, and we all get in trouble sometimes, and we all feel (really) bad sometimes. It's a part of life. Don't fight it—accept it, dust yourself off, and get up again.

Number four was I want people to be fair to me. Well, in an ideal fantasy world where war still has to be invented there would be no bad people, and everyone would be fair to everyone. This however is not the world we live in, and this gives us the choice of accepting the way things really are or trying to control the uncontrollable and losing our valuable energy in the process.

If you gave this statement a score of three or higher, please try to accept that this is just a part of life. A part that doesn't feel so good, but a mosquito bite doesn't feel great either and that too is a part of life.

Whatever happens—it is okay.

Number five was about relationships (friends, love, and family), I often get upset when the other person doesn't do what I want. This is a tricky one since this would make you the dominant person in the relationship. Trying to control everything and wanting everything to be perfect often means you want other people to do what you want. Even Frank, the nice guy who tried to please everyone wanted people to do what he wanted and got upset when they didn't. He wanted them to like him, and when they didn't, he got upset.

This too is an expectation that is set too high. Other people will do what they do, and that is okay. You can try to fight it and you can try to control their behavior with a variety of psychological techniques like the guilt trap[1], but it will only make you more and more disappointed.

Number six was I want to be in perfect health at all times, no aches, no pains, and no special symptoms. I used to get a full five on this one. Whenever I felt something out of the ordinary, I was sure it was some kind of cancer, a tropical disease, or something else that would eventually kill me.

Before I continue on this topic, let me tell you something funny. At the time I'm writing this book, I haven't had a

---

[1] The guilt trap typically manifests in statements like If you love me, you will...

special ache, pain, or any special symptom (no colds, flu, or headaches) for over a year. I'm not lying—this is the truth. After 2004, when my anxiety was gone, I still had colds and little things like that; well now even those are gone. My secret, without going into detail here since that would be a different book, is that I totally dropped consumption of sugar in any form. I don't even eat fruit anymore. If you're sick quite often, I highly recommend the book *Never Be Sick Again*, written by Raymond Francis. By the way, please don't replace sugar with artificial sweeteners. They will give you panic attacks and might actually make you sick. Simply search for excitotoxins and Dr. Russel Blaylock on the Web, and you'll learn why.

Our body is the most amazing machine you will ever see. It does everything it can to keep us alive, even when we don't always treat it the way we should. Have you ever seen the effect on a car engine when sugar is poured into the gas tank? It cannot function anymore and makes weird noises before dying.

If you then see what kind of things we put in our own engine, our body, it is amazing to learn how it deals with everything. Chemicals like alcohol, artificial sweeteners, taste enhancers, artificial coloring, soaps with sodium laureth sulfate in it, toothpaste with the toxic compound fluoride in it, and so on are all very bad for our body. Despite all this it keeps us alive and gets these things out.

But it won't do this without a struggle, and this struggle can in fact cause the symptoms you feel during a panic attack. I'll devote an entire chapter to this later on but I'll tell you this:

Our body is constantly communicating to us what it likes and what it dislikes.

It does this by giving aches and pains or by giving you the I-feel-great feeling.

If you use, consume, or smell things the body doesn't like, it will give you certain symptoms. Did you ever smell something that made you nauseated right away? That's your body saying, "Don't even think about eating that," and it communicates about everything you do to and for it.

So you will never be 100 percent symptom free because there's always something it wants to tell you. Don't fear aches and pains; instead consider them a powerful message from your body meant to guide and help you.

You'll get more on this in the chapter about foods.

Number seven was when I have an upcoming event, I plan ahead and imagine what it will be like. Doing this will give you anticipatory anxiety. I used to do this all the time. I would have been a good recruit for the CIA since I planned every possible outcome and every possible thing that might happen.

When my niece was about to have her wedding, she asked me to speak in front of the church. I had been lying awake for weeks because of this. Thinking about the possible panic attack I might have, what if I feel nauseated, what if I faint, or what if I need to leave. A what-if phrase will quite often be followed by anxiety. The exceptions are what if I win the lottery…but if you think about most of the what-if phrases you use, you'll see they can only make you anxious. They are the first domino that falls before a panic attack, and they can indeed keep you up all night or give you a nervous feeling all day.

The funny thing about this is that the actual situation will most often be different than any of the outcomes you've imagined. It's in fact another example of trying to control the uncontrollable. And it's a waste of time.

I used to prepare for everything and while I anticipated, I forgot to live my life; I forgot to actually enjoy the moment before the thing I had to do. The weeks before that wedding, I was so stressed that I didn't do anything fun at all because of a four-minute speech in front of a church. When I knew I had an important meeting, I would clear my schedule the days before, and I made sure I couldn't be sick, etc. Again, I forgot to live. And those events always turned out differently anyways.

It's okay to anticipate life-changing events like your own wedding, for instance. But when you start to anticipate something every week, you will be stressed each and every day, and you will forget to live.

Here, the whatever happens—it is okay credo will help again. Just let things come to you and deal with them when they happen. So when you have an anticipatory thought about anything, and when you feel you get anxious because of it, tell yourself **I will deal with this when it happens not now.**

There was a movie star who taught me this in 2004. He had an upcoming interview on national television and when asked if he was worried about the questions, he said, "I'll see what I say when I say it." What an amazing way of looking at life. When bad things happen, and they will for all of us at some point, we'll deal with it when it happens and not before.

Just imagine what life would feel like if you could live it like this. I personally still fall into the anticipation trap sometimes, but I quickly recover when I say, "I'll deal with it if and when it happens."

Are there things you worry about these days that you could apply this to?

It won't be easy! Intrusive worry-filled thoughts are persistent, but when you keep reminding them that you'll deal with them when they happen, they can't continue to harm you.

If you start with a what if, and you immediately block it, you'll have very light anxiety. If you allow it to continue, and you start to dwell on it, then you will feel the full load of anxiety. So it's always better to keep blocking those thoughts off than to allow them.

Number eight was I worry about losing control of myself, my thoughts, or my actions. This might not concern you, but it will be an interesting read anyway so please bear with me.

Some of my clients were afraid they would lose control while holding a knife, driving their car, or doing something else.

They thought they were going to harm themselves or other people. I'm not a psychologist, but as long as they are afraid of those things, it's simply the little anxiety devil that is playing with them. If they really wanted to harm themselves or other people it would be another story of course.

Try not to think about a purple elephant right now; you know, the one that would be used in cartoons. Are you trying not to think about that purple elephant? Well, you've just seen a flash of a purple elephant, haven't you? It's the same with the people that face this problem when they especially don't want to think about something like harming themselves or others. They think something weird and inappropriate and that thought scares them. "Oh my, is something wrong with me?" they think. So they really try not to think of it anymore…only to have that thought haunting them for as long as they are afraid of it.

The trick to stop this is again the idea that whatever happens—it is okay. Don't try to fight it because the more you do, the more it will haunt you. If you take away your fear of it, it will come up for a couple of weeks or months at the most and will then slowly vanish.

Number nine was I get irritated when things don't go as planned. This is about getting mad. Some people get mad when they lose control and when they feel things aren't going as planned. Getting mad and feeling that emotion is in fact a big stressor. Have you ever noticed that when you are mad your heart is pounding like crazy and that you are all tensed? That is okay if it happens once or twice a year. Some people however will have rated number nine as a five. They have anxiety issues because of this. The fact that they get mad over little things will cause a fatigued nervous system, and the nervous system that is worn down will in turn make it easier for them to get mad. This is a vicious circle.

The trick always lies in how you talk to yourself. When you get mad, you're saying things to yourself that will make you madder. If, however, you question those things, you can take it away. A good question for instance is "Can I really solve this problem if I get mad?" If the answer is yes, it is okay to get mad; if it is no, it is not okay to be mad. It will always be no.

Number ten was when I know I cannot control something and when other people are in control, I feel anxious. The best example of this is riding in the passenger seat of a car. You are not in control, and you do not decide the outcome. Sometimes a simple relationship can be an example of this as well. The partner will control your heart and your emotions. Some people don't like this and try to run away from it or control it. This is another one of the examples of things you cannot control anyway, so try to let go.

Conclusion

I don't know if you're feeling it yet, but trying to control the uncontrollable can be a major source of stress. And since stress is an important cause of anxiety you should try to let things go that you cannot control anyway.

A friend of mine once had a terrible accident with his motorcycle. He was driving through a crossroad at high speed when a car pulled up from the left. He hit the hood of the car, flew in the air, and yelled "I can see my home from here." Okay, that last part isn't true, but it would have been funny.

He was wearing a helmet and a special suit, but I'm sure you would imagine that he broke a lot of bones. Well…he didn't, but he should have. After the accident I talked to him and asked him how he got away with it.

He told me that "most people tense up when they have an accident with their bike. They try to hold on, they try to control everything. They are so tensed that they actually hurt their muscles and bones. The minute I saw I couldn't evade that car anymore, I let go. I let go of the handlebar, and I gave myself to the accident. I wasn't trying to avoid it, I wasn't trying to control it, and it was all okay. The doc told me that because of this, because my muscles where in such a relaxed state, I was like a cat, and I came down in a 'comfortable' manner."

Now obviously this result is not at all typical, but I believe it's a good metaphor for life in general. When you look around, might it be possible that the people who try to control everything are not in control at all? Not even in control of themselves? Is it possible that the people who live with a whatever happens—it's okay mentality are in fact happy and have great lives? I'm not trying to convince you here. Please have a look around and decide for yourself whether this is true or not. I'll talk more about this in a later chapter. But now, it is time for the main method of this book—the Tsunami Method®

Before I get to that method I want to point out that you'll get additional videos and articles on this "control" topic when you subscribe to my weekly tips newsletter on www.ilovepanicattacks.com/book/.

The Tsunami Method®

The Method to Stop Panic Attacks

The goal of this method is to help you to deal with a panic attack when you have one. Later chapters about foods, etc. will help you to prevent a panic attack; the previous chapter about control will help to prevent panic attacks, as well. The chapter after this one covers whatever happens—it's okay and will be the nuclear bomb to prevent panic attacks. But what can you do when the panic attack is already on you and wants to show you his powers?

In general:

The more you fight it, the worse it will get. The more you let go, the faster it will pass.

Before I explain the Tsunami Method®, I'll tell you how I discovered it. Imagine that you are swimming in the ocean; you're enjoying the sunshine, the fish around you (dolphins, whales, sharks, and squid ☺), and you are quite far from the shore. All of a sudden the weather changes, and a huge storm is there. There is a big twenty-foot Tsunami wave coming toward you. You don't know what to do, so you panic. You try to fight it; you try to swim away from it as fast as you can. The wave still catches you, takes you all the way up to its crest, and then pushes you deep under the water in a whirl of currents. Forty-five seconds later you arrive on the surface again, and you're so exhausted that you don't have the energy to swim to shore anymore. I'll end my story here because this is obviously a bad ending.

It doesn't have to end like this.

Imagine you're in the ocean and that wave is coming toward you. You say to yourself, "Wow, what a wave. I wish I had my camera with me. This would look good as my desktop wallpaper." At that point you realize there is no escape, and whatever you do, that wave will come, get you, take you up, and then push you under the water. So be it. You decide to accept this and stay calm. Forty-five seconds later, you come back to the surface, and you fill your lungs with fresh air. There was no panic attack, only some moderate anxiety, so you still have plenty of energy available to swim back to shore.

Can you imagine these things to be true? This is how you can stop a panic attack. The more you fight it, the more you will lose energy; the more you strain your nervous system, the more you'll be prone to having another attack. So the solution lies in the acceptance, in not fighting it.

Have you ever in your life waited on a jumping board above a pool, deciding whether you would jump or not? If you've ever done this, you probably were anxious when it was a jump of some distance. That anxiety is normal. Now if you did jump, the second you did it you accepted everything that was about to happen. In a way you said, "Whatever happens—it's okay," and you just went for it. It is this acceptance that is the solution for panic attacks.

Fear of the fear is cause number one of a panic attack. If you say, "Okay come and get me" to whatever you are afraid of, the fear is gone. It's that simple.

I talk for almost an hour about this subject on the first CD of my CD course you can get on ilovepanicattacks.com, but here are some important things you can do to accept instead of fight everything.

1. **Realize that you are afraid. That it's simply some anxiety you are feeling.**
2. **Try to see why you are anxious.**
3. **Accept it and laugh with it.**
4. **Start floating.**

Realize that you are afraid. That it's simply some anxiety you are feeling.

I didn't even realize I had panic attacks the first couple of years I had them. I didn't know this was anxiety, and I didn't know I had the power to make it worse with my own thoughts. I thought there was something really wrong with me that had nothing to do with anxiety. I was wrong.

When you simply tell yourself "Okay, I'm anxious, and I can make it worse if I use scary phrases now," you're one step ahead already. It sounds too easy, but really, the next time that you are anxious or are in the middle of a panic attack, tell yourself (out loud whenever possible) "I am anxious."

Try to See Why You Are Anxious

This will take some practice, but why is it that you are anxious? Quite often there is a specific factor. There are 1001 factors, but the most common ones are:

- I'm somewhere without an immediate exit.
- I'm not supposed to leave here.
- What are people going to think of me?
- I'm in my car.
- I'm in a supermarket / a restaurant / a theater.
- I'm in a plane.
- There are too many people here.
- I'm all alone here.
- There is something wrong with me. Am I going to die?

Try to pinpoint what it is the cause for you. There can be external factors (99 percent of this list are external factors) or internal factors (being afraid of symptoms that you are feeling or things you feel going on in your body).

Explain this cause to yourself, explain why you are feeling it, and do it in the friend-method way. Explain it in a calming way just as you would explain it to a friend who was scared. This is a very important step. When you explain to yourself why you are anxious, something strange will happen. Try it. Don't focus on all the symptoms or feelings, focus on this phrase "I am anxious right now because…"

Accept It and Laugh with It

Do not try to fight the anxious feeling, simply accept it. This is another very important key to a life without panic attacks, but it's the one that is very difficult to explain. I promise you that if you accept the anxiety, over time it will go away. This breaks the fear of the fear cycle, and when you truly master this, it will only take a couple of weeks to have no panic attacks anymore. I do admit, however, that this is not an easy task, and you will really have to keep practicing it until you master it. But I did it, and the thousands of clients who have bought my CD course on ilovepanicattacks.com have done it. If we can do it, you can do it, too.

So accepting it is important, and the best way to do this is simply to tell yourself "I accept this anxiety and the feelings I have."

Laughing with it can also help a lot. The reason is this gives a very strong message to your body that the panic system was not needed. If you were ever in real danger, e.g., in the woods with a real tiger in front of you, you would never ever start to laugh. So when you DO laugh or use humor, it is in fact a powerful defense mechanism.

When I had my vertigo and dizzy spells, I would tell myself, "Look here, I can get drunk, and I don't even need any alcohol. I can still drive, the cops can pull me over, and everything will be fine—GREAT."

Whatever you can think of will do. And for symptoms you'll have to look hard to find a humorous phrase, but you will always find something. Try to sit down with a piece of paper in front of you beforehand. When the panic attack is already there, you won't find anything because of the little blackout you will have.

Another trick to use humor is to picture yourself in a soap opera and see yourself from the camera's perspective having that panic attack in the funniest way possible while the audience laughs. That one helped me and many of my clients.

Start Floating. This is a technique I read about in Dr. Claire Weekes's book, called *Self Help for Your Nerves,* and I've further developed it. Imagine you are in a little boat on the Niagara River. You can start to paddle; you can start to do whatever you want, but we both know what will eventually happen. If you decide to let yourself float and to "give yourself" to the situation, you are much more powerful.

Plus, floating is a very relaxing thing to do. Few people get very nervous in a bathtub, for instance; most people can really relax when they float around in water. The trick here is to imagine yourself floating through your problem, through the thing you've defined as causing your anxiety right now.

So whenever you are anxious, use abdominal breathing and start to imagine that you are floating through your problems. Don't fight them and don't resist; instead say, "Come and get me. Show me what you've got," and start to float. It takes some practice, but you will feel this is a very powerful step to stop panic attacks.

The abdominal breathing by the way is powerful. To test what this is, lie down somewhere and put one hand on your stomach and the other hand on your chest. When you breathe, only the hand on your stomach should move up and down. That's when you know you are doing this right.

Every animal breathes through the abdomen when in a relaxed state. High breathing (nonabdominal breathing) is used when oxygen is needed quickly when the animal is in danger. So by breathing through the abdomen, you are communicating I am not in any danger. When you try this in an anxious situation, you might notice that your heart will start to pound even faster for a couple of seconds. Don't worry about this, this is normal, and means you will calm down.

Conclusion

These are some very important steps to my Tsunami Method®. I have created a video about this that will be sent to you in a couple of weeks if you've visited www.ilovepanicattacks.com/book/ and subscribed to the mailing and video list.

This method is really powerful, but it will take some practice on your part. There is no magic pill or a magic cure that will work in twenty-four hours. Believing that will keep you looking for the Holy Grail for the rest of your life. This method will take a couple of weeks or even months to show you its full capacity, but I promise it can give you the result you've been looking for. The best side effect is that this result will actually last.

The next step is to write the four bullet points down on a piece of paper that you carry with you. Read and execute them during a panic attack and keep practicing. After a panic attack, when you're back home, write down what you could have said to yourself for each step. Try to do this exercise because chances are that your mental abilities during the attack will be limited. This is very normal because all your energy will be used to prepare a good fight or a good run that will never happen.

I've learned this when I was studying the astronauts at the NASA that fly the space shuttle. They are obviously very intelligent people, but they still have to practice some basic handling in the cockpit over and over again. "When the space shuttle gives this error message, you should push buttons A, G, and T." Simple…but they keep practicing things like this. The reason is that whenever they have a "Houston, we have a problem" situation, they might panic, and their minds might go blank. The only thing they will know then is what they've been practicing over and over again.

You go through the same sequence when you have moderate anxiety or a major panic attack, and this is the reason why you should practice the Tsunami method® before and after panic attacks as much as you can. It's the only way to feel its full power and see how easily it can stop a panic attack if you've practiced. It's a bit like karate. You need to train to get your black belt, and when you have it, you'll be able to defend yourself wherever and whenever. When you're still working to get your black belt, you'll already be able to use a lot of your defensive power but not all of it.

Please take the time to write the 4 steps down now before you continue your reading.

"Whatever Happens—
It's Okay"

And How This Can Improve Your Life in Funny Ways

In my CD course, the main and most important phrase is "Whatever happens—it is okay." It's so important that I even registered it as a tagline. The reason is simple. A person who truly believes this phrase has no anxiety at all. This is someone who can jump out of a plane without a parachute and think, "Whatever happens—it is okay." Now obviously, you don't need to become that person, but that's how powerful this is.

It was 2004 and I was in the States, overcoming my own panic issues. There were some wildfires in California (where I was), and I was watching the news on a local TV station. The camera crew followed a woman as she returned to her home. They walked up a hill and saw that everything was gone. The entire area was black, and where her house used to be, you could only see debris.

"So what is this?" asked the journalist while he pointed to a couple of large chunks of melted metal.

"Those were my classic cars…Porsches, Cadillac,s etc.," said the woman. "They were not insured for this."

It was immediately interesting to see how upbeat she was.

"Isn't this hard for you? You seem so calm about this," said the interviewer.

"Yeah," replied the woman. "I could start to cry right now, but what good is that going to do? What happened has happened, and now it's up to me to deal with it. It's all okay."

That was one of the most amazing interviews I had ever seen at the time. I can only imagine how I would have reacted in her situation. My tears would have been able to put out the entire fire.

She gave a very important secret of life. When bad things happen, accept them, deal with them, and move on. The alternative—getting knocked down and staying down—is much worse.

On top of this, anxious people will continuously anticipate bad events even before they happen. I know I did, as did every single client I've ever had.

Do Not Anticipate Bad Things.

To our body and mind, vividly imagining things is the same as them happening in real time. So if you anticipate that something bad is going to happen, your body will go through the same emotions as if it really happened. That's why a vivid nightmare can wake you up all anxious with every symptom that you would have had if the dream were to be real.

So by anticipating that bad thing we fear actually happens each and every time we think of it. Over and over again, like an endless loop of bad emotions.

In the end, it's better not to anticipate at all and have it happen for real. At least it only happens once then. That's another good thing to tell yourself when you're anticipating. But the best thing to tell yourself is without a single doubt "Whatever happens—it is okay. I will deal with it when it happens not now." This phrase can stop stress and anxiety before it can harm or touch you. And you can use it whenever you are anxious. It uses the powerful technique of acceptance. You accept that the bad thing you fear will happen to you and t that is okay.

I haven't had a panic attack since 2004, but I still remember an anxious moment I had in 2007. I got a serious allergy in my eyes because they didn't want to tolerate contact lenses any longer. I had very bad vision and glasses were not comfortable for me because the lenses were so thick they actually were bulletproof. So I was thinking about Lasik eye surgery. On the Web I read all the horror stories from people who had a bad outcome. Some even went blind. That was tricky, but I decided to go through with it under the approach that whatever happens—it is okay.

The day of the operation I was lying down on the operating table, and my heart started to race. I was anxious. "What if it fails and five minutes from now, I'm blind? I would always regret having made this decision. You can still run away, Geert." Those were my thoughts. Here too, I could calm myself down with the whatever happens phrase. I actually accepted that going blind would be okay. It immediately calmed me down.

Two things were very important in this situation:

- I actually had to believe that it really was okay, even though I would prefer not to go blind, of course.

- I had to say it to myself, and if necessary, I would have to keep repeating it. It is better to continue to block a bad thought off with a phrase like this than to accept the bad thought and let it get through and change your emotions.

And it worked. I was calm and I can still see 20/20 today in both eyes.

Can you feel the power of this phrase? Every time you think what if, you can actually use it. And yes, I do realize this means thinking things like if I crash my car, that would be okay or if I die, that would be okay. I know it might not be okay, but these are choices you will have to make. If you want to calm down and live life with a smile on your face and virtually no anxiety, this is how you will have to learn to think. Magical things will start to happen.

Accept everything—play with that phrase and IF the bad thing really happens, THEN you can deal with it. There's no point in living that bad moment over and over again in your thoughts. WHEN it happens, you'll deal with it. Only then but not beforehand. Otherwise it's as if you're living that movie *Groundhog Day* from 1993, where every day is the previous day repeating itself over and over again.

I promise you this is a very powerful technique, and I sincerely hope you will start to play with it. Amazing things will happen, and you'll see yourself doing things with a smile again that you never imagined doing.

In the next chapter we'll start to prevent panic attacks altogether by stabilizing your body.

Foods and Other Things That Can Cause Anxiety

And Why Big Corporations Don't Like You

This chapter is one of the most important chapters in this book. It contains breakthrough secrets that will help to prevent panic attacks and anxiety. If I didn't know what I'm about to share with you here, I would still have panic attacks.

I am not a doctor, but I can only hope that doctors will start sharing this information with their patients as soon as possible. (Some like Dr. Mercola and Dr. Russell Blaylock already do.)

Bart had a problem. He was dizzy and nauseated for a couple of hours every day. Bart was an entrepreneur with a company that has over one million dollars in profits every year, so this was really starting to harm his career and his bottom line.

He went to see his physician who ran some blood tests. Everything was perfectly fine. So Bart had a brain scan done in the hospital to check for anomalies like a tumor. This too turned out negative.

Although Bart was relieved, it actually worried him even more. If there was nothing to be seen, maybe he had a disease that was so new there wouldn't be a cure for it.

A friend of Bart had already followed my CD course on ilovepanicattacks.com and showed him the Web site. For Bart, this was worth a shot since he really wanted to find the solution. Around week four, the week about ingredients and foods that do weird things to the body, Bart's life started to change. He had to give up some things he did every day, but about two weeks later, I got an e-mail from him that the dizziness and the nausea were completely gone. They never returned.

I could give you stories for a couple of hours, but I'll limit it to just a final one on this topic.

Maggie had a problem, too. Every time she sat down in her car, she started to shake, had difficulty focusing on the other cars, and it felt as if she wasn't herself., She felt as if she was floating out of her own body. The same happened when she traveled by plane or by boat.

She got very anxious every time this happened and decided to avoid these places as much as she could. Every time she was in her car or in a plane, it would happen. Maggie thought it was because of the car or the plane, but she failed to see there was this one thing she did right before she sat down in the car or the plane…that was actually causing the symptoms.

It took me a long time myself to find this one. As I said earlier, our bodies will continuously communicate to us what they like, what they don't like, and so on. When you have a certain symptom and your physician can't find anything, chances are your body is trying to tell you something about a thing you eat/drink/smell or apply to your skin. There are obvious examples and there are less obvious examples.

Here are some obvious ones:

-        You get bitten by a poisonous snake. Thirty minutes later, your heart starts to race, and you feel dizzy and nauseous. There is venom in your body, and your body is trying to tell you that, just in case you missed the snakebite and paid no attention to it.

-        You drink a lot of alcohol. At first you feel lightheaded, and you're a bit dizzy. The next morning, you have a dry mouth and a serious headache and nausea.

These two are obvious, and they might not give you any anxiety or panic because you clearly know why you are feeling all those things. That said, this shows that when some things get into our blood stream (like venom or alcohol), we get strange sensations. And if these two can do that, other things can do the same thing.

Here are some less obvious examples:

-        The panic system gives you the fight-or-flight response and speeds your entire body up by giving you an adrenalin rush. Caffeine (found in coffee and tea, for instance) mimics this and speeds our entire body up. This might not be news to you since so many people use it to stay awake in the morning. That said, it does much more than that. Caffeine can give you the following symptoms: nausea, headache, dry mouth, and sweating; it can also make you more prone to illness like colds. Caffeine is in fact a pro-oxidant. Where an antioxidant protects you and slows you down, caffeine turns everything up a notch, and makes you live and age faster. People like us do not need this; we can be nervous without caffeine and adding caffeine will make us more anxious. It will make us worry about little things that don't matter at all. Tea is in the same boat. Tea contains healthy antioxidants, but in the tea leaves you'll find caffeine that can give you a whole range of strange sensations that can lead to anxiety. Try to stay away from both for a couple of weeks; by then you'll feel the difference, and you won't return to them. One cup of coffee a day is too much. If I drank one cup of coffee a day, I would still have anxiety and panic attacks. It's not worth it. If you drink more than two cups a day, try to stop on a Friday since you will have a headache for a couple of days.

- Aspartame is a very tricky one. I won't go into too much detail here, but Dr. Russell Blaylock has done some amazing studies on this artificial sweetener. It gave me severe headaches, dizziness, and nausea. I also got aches and pains in my entire body like I had the flu. It starts to change the firing of the neurons in your brain, and when that happens, you can start to shake, experience nausea, headache, and a whole other range of problems simply because you drank a diet drink or chewed some chewing gum. Try to look into this and check everything you eat for this ingredient. Real sugar isn't good either, but it is a whole lot better than this one.

And if you think aspartame helps you to lose weight, think again. It actually makes you crave more calories afterward. It's not worth it. Other artificial sweeteners like sucralose are a little less bad, but they will give you intestinal and other problems. Try to stay away from them for at least a couple of weeks, so I can prove my point.

- Monosodium glutamate (MSG) is one of the most frequently used taste enhancers since the fifties. It causes the same problems in the brain that aspartame does and then some more. I talk a lot more about this on the Web site if you need more information on it; please, stay away from this one and look for the other names the smart food manufacturers try to give it now that they know more and more people don't want to eat it any longer. Other ingredients that quite often contain or are MSG are hydrolyzed soy protein, dextrose, sodium caseinate, yeast extract, gelatin, and glutamic acid. Trying to ban this one from your meals will be difficult at first, but once that you find the brands that are okay, you can stick to them.

A good rule of thumb is that everything that was manufactured in a factory (instant soups, luncheon meats, sauces, and other things you add to enhance taste) is suspicious. Things you create from scratch yourself will usually be fine. Fresh vegetables and fresh meat will always be fine, as long as you don't add any taste enhancers (sauces and some herb mixes that contain MSG).

- Chemicals in general can give you weird sensations because they can poison you. Fresh paint, that new car smell, and air fresheners can make you nauseated and/or make you dizzy, give you a headache, and can even give you a fever sometimes. So if you specifically get weird sensations in your car, the off-gassing from the plastics in there might be causing your problem, especially if it is a new car. In Maggie's case her additional problem was she always drank some coffee to calm her stomach before getting into the car or the plane, and the opposite happened.

So these smells are important. When you feel weird or bad somewhere, think about the smell. Was there one? If it doesn't smell natural, it is chemical, and it will give some people (us) symptoms.

-        Things we apply on our skin are very important as well. Let's start with the fluoride you'll find in most toothpaste. Even if you don't swallow it, it still gets into your bloodstream because of the very thin layer of skin you have in your mouth. It can give you that floating feeling, as if you're not really yourself, plus a variety of other things. If you suffer from panic attack symptoms, it's worth it to find one without fluoride. Quite often the organic ones will help you out. I've been using them for a couple of years now, and I still don't have any cavities, so they still protect your teeth very well. They will actually protect your breath better than the chemical ones because they don't disrupt the delicate balance in your mouth.

Shower gels and soaps are important, too. They contain ingredients like sodium laureth sulfate. This is a very toxic chemical and because it is not ingested, people used to think it is okay. Our skin is made up out of living cells that "eat" what we put on them. Just below is our blood, and things that we put on our skin will get in there, especially when the skin is thin.

I don't want to be the hippy guy that says everything is bad for you. But since you have anxiety and panic attacks, I would like to suggest that if you have weird symptoms you do not like, try to switch to 100 percent organic body gels and soaps, shampoos, and even deodorants for a couple of weeks to see if you feel a difference.

I'll end the chapter on the ingredients, foods, and odors that cause panic and anxiety symptoms right here; if you're interested in this subject, I talk a lot more about this in the CD course you can find on the Web site (ilovepanicattacks.com).

Moving Your Body and Why This Alone Prevents Panic Attacks and Anxiety

Working out is good for us—you've heard that a million times. What you might not have heard is that working out too much is not so good for us. Chances are, however, that you don't belong to the category of people who work out too much.

Moving your body can help prevent panic attacks, and it can help while you are having a panic attack. Although you've heard of the importance of working out before, please bear with me because this is an important chapter.

Mark had a certain problem. He was not an anxious type and all was well when he was at home or somewhere outside. For him, problems began whenever he was inside, especially when there were a lot of people present. Five minutes after arriving at a concert, a restaurant or anywhere else, he would have to sit or stand. Mark would get some strange sensations. He felt like he was going to lose consciousness, and his heart started to race. It was as if there wasn't enough oxygen in the air or something. He never fainted, but often he had to run out of the venue, and this was becoming a problem.

After Mark had followed the CD course, he told me his problem was gone. The main things that helped him were the advice on the foods and the advice on working out.

Our body is an amazing machine. I'm sure you've found this out. I'm quite a fan of everything it does and can do. Whenever something bad happens, it tries to make sure that thing won't happen again. Giving you anxiety beforehand is one of those mechanisms.

But there's another one. Suppose you haven't worked out in three months or longer and just suppose we go running together. How long would it take before you'd have a:

- racing heart
- out-of-breath feeling
- sweat attack
- mild to major nausea

Not long probably, and it wouldn't really scare you, I guess. You know why it is happening, so it all would be okay.

Now why are these symptoms there? To run, to use any muscle, that muscle needs to burn energy, and just like a fire needs oxygen to burn, your muscles need it too. They will be screaming for oxygen in fact. As a result, your heart starts to pound faster to move the oxygen in your blood as quickly as it can to your muscles; you get out of breath because the muscles demand too much oxygen—more than you can give them. All the energy production makes you hot, so you start to sweat. The digestion is not so important, so it stops, and food sitting in your stomach might make you nauseous.

The oxygen part is important here. When there is an oxygen problem you will start to feel lightheaded, something you might have felt before when working out or running. Your body will remember this and will try to make everything more efficient for the next time you put your body through this. That's why, when you continue to work out, your body will always need less and less oxygen to do the same thing. If you haven't worked out for a long time, your body is not fuel-efficient. It needs a lot of oxygen to do minor things. Gradually this gets better until you can actually run and still hold a normal conversation. Amazing, right?

Okay. So if you do not have a good conditioning of the body, if it is not oxygen efficient, panic attacks and problems might arise.

Each time Mark went into a room filled with people, his body quickly noticed there was less oxygen in there than outside. (That's normal because other people are using the oxygen, so it is shared between everyone.) When the "not-enough-oxygen" alarm goes off, his heart rate goes up (to spread the available oxygen as fast as possible); he starts to breath faster, and he might start to sweat or might feel nauseated, dizzy etc. It's exactly as if he was running—it's the exact same system. But because he isn't running he worries about this a lot and starts the panic attack cycle.

This is the most important reason why working out is very important. When you do, your body will get oxygen efficient, and whenever you are in a low-oxygen situation, you won't even feel it. It will know how to deal with this and all will be okay. Is that good enough of a reason to start working out? I hope so.

The second reason is that it will create a better balance in your brain chemicals like serotonin. In short, it will put a smile on your face.

This has some weird consequences. Just imagine you've won the lottery (a couple of million dollars), and you have the winning ticket in your back pocket. You stand in line somewhere, and there are a lot of people, and you are nauseated and dizzy. I might be wrong, but is it possible that that thought of the winning ticket in your pocket is going to make everything okay? That it will be easier to say "Whatever happens—it is okay. I have the winning ticket in my back pocket, so I don't care about anything"? Well that's what working out will do for you; you'll have that ticket with you at all times. I am not a scientist, and I don't fully understand why this happens, but people who work out are more stable, less anxious, and definitely less depressed.

For this reason, I strongly suggest your start a workout routine. Here are some important things to keep in mind:

-   Choose cardio over weights. It's the oxygen efficiency that needs to improve; your muscle growth is less important

-   Work out at least two times a week (preferably three times) and do it for twenty minutes. The pace must make you breathe faster. A simple walk is not okay and won't do much.

-   Before starting any workout regimen, always talk to your physician and get his okay, especially if it's been a long time since you really moved your body a lot.

-   Do not use sport drinks, sport shakes, or sport bars. They quite often contain aspartame or sucralose and always contain a lot of chemicals. They are not good for you.

- Try to work out in the open air whenever possible. Working out on a treadmill in your house is fine. (I do it in front of the television sometimes.) But open windows to let a flow of fresh air in if you work out indoors. In-house air is filled with not so super things like dust and off-gassed chemicals. When you work out outside, don't do it near a big road or freeway with a lot of polluting cars.

- Do not overdo it. Too much of a good thing is bad for you, and you'll notice that professional athletes run in trouble with injuries and other problems at some point in their life. Three times a week for twenty minutes is enough, as long as it is a vigorous exercise.

It will take a couple of weeks, but I promise you will feel better in all areas of your life. They have done tests on depressed people who could not stay depressed when put on a workout regimen. It does wonders for anxiety, too, and will give you that feel-good feeling.

What Other People think of You

And Why You Shouldn't Care

Most people spend a large part of their life worrying about what other people think of them. Quite a lot of them even change their actions to "please" other people. I know I did.

A large part of my anxiety was in fact caused by this way of thinking. When I sat down in a restaurant and got nauseated, it wasn't that I was so scared I would actually throw up. I was scared other people would see it and think I was weird. The same with driving my car; driving somewhere all alone was usually fine, but the minute other people were involved in their cars, my anxiety started.

I was brought up believing "what will people think of you if you're not…or when you…" My mother cared a lot about what other people thought of me. Most mothers do that and this is probably okay, but I took it with me as an adolescent and later on as an adult.

Being a hypersensitive person, I could also feel what other people were feeling about themselves and also about me. Like a chameleon, I started to adapt so they would like me or so I could blend in. Have you ever done this? I also had a feeling of guilt every time I had to use the word *no* to let someone down. I didn't like that feeling, so I used *yes* much more often. The problem was I was placing everyone else above myself, and I forgot the most important person I would ever meet— me.

I also noticed how fatiguing it was to adapt myself all the time. I used this analogy before, but it's as if you work for the CIA, and you must continuously scan for terrorists. I did that all the time, trying to read other peoples' minds to see what they thought of me.

A part of the solution for my own panic attacks was the whatever they think—it is okay credo. The minute I didn't care anymore about doing something stupid with my car, myself, or something else in front of other people, I could actually relax. It's was as if a giant weight had been lifted off my shoulders since there were no expectations anymore.

What are the things you do because other people want you to? Or worse, what are the things you do because you THINK other people want you to? You should make a list of these things because you'll find out you do this more often than you think. Knowing who the culprits are is the first part of the solution.

I've talked about this before, but some people will always hate you, some people will always like you, and some people will always be in between. So the whatever they think—it is okay credo is again a powerful phrase.

If you like this subject, you'll get more info on this in the on Web site ilovepanicattacks.com.

Reprogramming Your Mind for Success and Less Anxiety or Stress

Did I already mention our bodies are amazing things? I'm sure I did a million times. The amygdala, the emotional part of our brain, is another one of these amazing things. It remembers emotions and tries to regulate our behavior based on things it remembers. If you ever got hurt in a relationship, the amygdala remembers. When your new partner does something that your old partner did right before hurting you, the alarm will start to sound.

If you ever had a panic attack somewhere, and you had a lot of anxiety as a result, your amygdala will remember this and when you are in a location that resembles (or is) the old location where you had the panic attack, it will give you anxiety, so you stay away from that thing or event. This was a very strong defense mechanism 500 years ago. If you ever met a big black wolf in a dark hole somewhere in the woods, thanks to the amygdala you would start to run when next you saw another dark hole somewhere else.

The problem, however, begins when you've had an anxious feeling that was inappropriate because there was nothing to be scared of. It will still commit to doing its job and will give you anxiety, fear, and a whole range of symptoms in the future, even when there was and is no real danger. At that point, it has already been conditioned to give you anxiety. You can change this by breaking the conditioning.

What is conditioning?

Ivan Pavlov discovered this when he did a little test on a dog. When you put food in front of a dog, the dog starts to salivate.

So what Pavlov did is while putting food in front of the dog, he would ring a little bell. The dog would start to salivate because of the food and would hear a bell. Pavlov repeated this setup a couple of times and then he rang the bell without putting food in front of the dog. The dog started to salivate. He had learned that the bell meant food was coming. This is conditioning.

Did you ever hear a song that you hadn't heard for a long time and feel the exact way you felt when you last heard that song? Advertisers use this principle a lot. They show happy people or something that you aspire to, and then they show their product or service with their logo. If they do this enough, you will already start to feel good simply thinking about or consuming their product or service. Now please don't think that wouldn't work on you. It really does.

Did you ever know someone you know was mad at you because they looked at you in a certain way? You knew this because you had been conditioned to know that when that look is there, a fight or a remark will follow. We are filled with these things in our brain (don't touch a pan after cooking because it is hot, people with… are dangerous, people with … are to be trusted). This kind of conditioning also happened when you had anxious moments and everything that happened around you when you had a panic attack is linked up to it.

I don't know if you've taken the time to see my video on ilovepanicattacks.com, but there I explain that I had a panic attack in an auditorium during an exam. A couple of weeks later, I was in the movie theater with my girlfriend, and my mind recognized the setting as the same setting as an auditorium. So from that moment on I got panic attacks in theaters.

That's how panic attacks can spread like a little virus. This is the reason why it is so important that you actually apply every technique I share with you in this book. You can only stop it by reprogramming your mind.

Reprogramming the Mind

Exposure therapy uses this concept. The psychologists who use this believe that by putting you in contact with what scares you, you will see that all is fine and this will reprogram your mind.

I am not a psychologist, but I disagree. When you have a panic attack, nothing real happens anyway, and still the panic attacks won't stop. When you put someone who's afraid of dogs in a park filled with dogs, that person will have a lot of anxious feelings, even though not a single dog barks at him or touches him. The link that dogs give me anxiety will, in fact, be reinforced.

What you need to learn first are tools to control your own anxiety, so you can use these tools in the moment of danger. That's how you can take anxiety away and that's how you can reprogram your mind. That is the goal of this book and that is also the goal of my CD course.

With the methods and techniques you get here, you go out and practice. At first you will still feel anxious. You need to accept this; it is very normal, and you have been programmed to feel this anxiety. Then you start to work on it with the techniques, and little by little, you learn that you can stop a panic attack, even when you are in the place that scared you or when you feel something in your body. This is when true change will occur. Little by little you will be reprogramming yourself and learn that it is safe to do this or that or to feel this or that.

If Pavlov had continued to ring his bell 100 times without giving food, by the end the dog wouldn't salivate at the sound. He would have learned that the bell doesn't mean anything. There is however one important remark. If Pavlov had rung the bell forty-one times, and just as the dog started to believe that the bell didn't mean food is coming, he brought food, then the dog would have learned a powerful lesson. He would have learned that even when there is no food for countless times, it might come back in the future, so he would keep hoping and salivating.

In anxiety terms this means that if you manage to do your thing again without anxiety, and one day you do feel anxious again, you are at an important and life-changing crossroad.

What side are you going to pick?

- "There you go. I knew it couldn't be gone. I'll have anxiety forever." Depression and a bad life will follow this thinking.

-        "You know what, I knew this would happen, and it is okay. I'll keep playing with it. Anxiety is a part of life, and as long as I remember how to deal with it, it can't win." A great life will follow this thinking.

This is an important distinction and an important lesson. There will always be some anxiety sometimes; one of the things I mentioned in the chapter about control is that it is unrealistic to expect life to be perfect at all times. It really isn't for anybody. People who let themselves slide at that point will go back to zero. People who decide that this is a part of life can keep it up.

My clients and I have had countless of opportunities to fall back into the trap because we felt something or because we were uncomfortable somewhere. We all chose to accept that feeling and remind ourselves that whatever happens—it is okay. That way you can continue to reprogram yourself for the better.

I hope you're ready for the challenge. You're getting close to the end of this book, and I want to emphasize again that reading it won't help you but using it will!

Reprogramming a broken record takes some time and devotion, but when it is done, when you keep working on it, you will be able to control yourself. Isn't that funny? By letting go of control with phrases like whatever happens—it is okay you actually gain control!

So the reprogramming part will work like this for you:

- You do the things that scare you.
- You feel anxious (that's normal), and you start to play with the methods you've learned in this book.
- You survive.
- Next time you go again, and you go through the same cycle, but you feel more confident already.
- You survive and start to think, "It wasn't THAT bad."
- Next time you go again…

And so on, until your amygdala and memory has learned that going there and doing this and that is actually fine. I might feel anxious, but it isn't going to harm me or change the outcome. At that point you will be FREE.

There is however one crucial element here: you do the things that scare you. This is a very difficult step because it means going out there and putting yourself in "danger" when you still have panic attacks. That's scary, I know, but we've all had to do it; it's the only way. The panic attacks won't go away until you take this necessary step. You can read all you want about how to drive a car, the only way to master it is to get in the car and do funny things with it like stalling (at first).

When I still had my panic attacks, I jumped on planes to look for a solution. Each time I sat on one of those planes, I had a severe panic attack, but I continued doing it because I knew that was the only way to find the solution. It's as if you stick your hand in a box full of fire, but you do it anyway because you know the key, the solution, is in there somewhere.

I'm still glad I did it, and if you want to look back on this moment in a couple of weeks, months, and years and be proud of how you managed to do the unthinkable and actually overcome your panic attacks, you'll have to jump into the deep part of the pool. You'll have to take this risk.

I hope you will do this. You owe it to yourself, and you will never regret it, however hard it will be.

I wish you all the best with these techniques. If you decide to use them, you will see results.

Good luck!

Geert – www.ilovepanicattacks.com

CPSIA information can be obtained at www.ICGtesting.com
Printed in the USA
244194LV00005B/135/P